Fabulosity Is You!

A Woman's Guide For Building Her Confidence, Fashion Tips, Weight Loss Tips, Skin Care Secrets, Relationships and Pursuing Her Purpose by Winsome Campbell-Green

Table of Contents

CHAPTER 1: S.E.X.Y DEFINED — 2

CHAPTER 2: STYLE IT! WORK IT! LOVE IT! — 8

CHAPTER 3: ENHANCE AND ACCENTUATE, BUT DON'T ALTER — 18

CHAPTER 4: GET WITH THE GLOW! — 22

CHAPTER 5: DO-IT-YOURSELF NATURAL SCRUBS AND MASKS THAT MAKE YOUR SKIN GLOW! — 30

CHAPTER 6: MAKE-UP: LESS IS MORE! — 38

CHAPTER 7: LOVE, RELATIONSHIPS AND HEARTBREAK — 46

CHAPTER 8: SECRETS TO A HAPPY MARRIAGE: CONFESSIONS OF A NEWLYWED — 54

CHAPTER 9: NOTHING IS AS SEXY AS A WOMAN WITH CONFIDENCE — 60

CHAPTER 10: WHIP THAT BODY IN SHAPE: EFFECTIVE EXERCISE PROGRAMS & ROUTINES THAT WORKS — 64

AUTHOR BIO — 71

THANK YOU FOR READING! — 72

Dear Readers:

This book is written specifically for you. The goal of this book is to help you build your confidence, empower you and it seeks to help you enhance what is already there. I want you to know I am no "expert" and the thoughts and opinions expressed here are based on my own experiences. As you read through each chapter, I hope you can examine the thoughts expressed through your own "filters." My hope is that you may walk away with some wisdom or insight that you did not previously consider. I also hope that you will become a woman who is bold enough to pursue her purpose.

    Winsome Campbell-Green

Copyright Fabulosity Is You! A Woman's Guide For Building Her Confidence, Fashion Tips, Weight Loss Tips, Skin Care Secrets, Relationships and Pursuing Her Purpose by Winsome Campbell-Green

All Rights reserved Winsome Campbell-Green © 2013

Chapter 1: S.E.X.Y Defined

- *Strong*
- *Empowered*
- *Xclusive*
- *Youthful*

You should be *strong* enough to learn from your mistakes, gather your strength from your struggles, and overcome every obstacle courageously. Be *empowered* to become agents of change within your society. Always be *xclusive* so you do not appear common and avoid the situations that do not serve your higher purpose. Embrace a healthy, happy and positive lifestyle that reflects in your physical appearance and you will be *youthful*. The word sexy appears in our life much more frequent. Almost everything around you is presented as alluring and sexy. The inner meaning conveys being *erotic and aroused* by something or someone. However, I do think it is a misunderstood word different people will use in different situations. For some people, *everything* is sexy; cars, food and the list are endless. On many occasions I have used the phrase with my husband when stating the obvious. In turn, he does the same. Many variations of the phrase exist. It behooves you to examine what *sexy* means to you. Overall it is a positive complimentary word when used in the right context.

    However, in today's society so many girls, and young women believe that being sexy means exposing private areas of the anatomy, perhaps to solicit compliments from the opposite sex. Everyone has a right to how they present themselves. However if you are trying to mold yourself as a woman of worth, consider the possibility that attention must be placed on what clothes you wear. It is unacceptable to have your bodyparts spilling out. If your objective is to be sexy, you don't need to have any part of your body showing at all. Remember the aim of the game is to become a woman of purpose and potential. To become a woman of worth you owe it to yourself to represent your image in the best possible light. You are always building your personal brand.

Over the years my own style has evolved. I can remember after leaving University my style did not change much from typical jeans and tanks. Of course nothing was wrong with the way I looked. However, I did have an image of how I wanted to dress, but felt it was not necessary for me to up the ante. I never tried to set trends, but my wardrobe was still very classy and stylish. My style also changed when I entered the corporate world of work. I thought many young women were allowing fashion get the best of them, by observing those around me. How you dress sends a strong message about who you are. What message are you trying to send to the world? Do not allow fashion to get the best of you! This is very serious and a somewhat troubling topic as so many women feel they must wear the latest trends to look good. Wrong! Ask yourself these questions the next time you reach for that 'color block' dress:

- Is it compatible with the climate you live in?
- Does the color compliment your undertone and body shape?
- Is it tailored to fit your body type?

- Are you comfortable?

Those are just some of my basic rules when shopping (depends on what I am looking for). If I am in doubt I keep it simple and I always make the right choice. Every woman has a particular style. I will explore this further in the next chapter and teach you some very effective techniques. There is no need to show off your endowments to feel or appear *sexy*. Love yourself and embrace your physical form. I do not believe in excesses and the simpler is always the better. Sophia Loren sums this up very nicely: *"A woman's dress should be like a barbed wire fence: serving its purpose without obstructing the view."* To begin building your confidence you must look in the mirror and appreciate yourself as you are. Start being comfortable and happy with yourself. In the next few chapters I will explore in detail simple, fun and inexpensive ways to look and feel like the Goddess that you are. The time is now to begin to claim your confidence and grow into a beautiful, and empowered woman. If you are newly single, feeling heartbroken, or divorced, it's not too late to get back your "fabulosity." You already have the beauty, and the intelligence, so let's begin the journey!

CHAPTER 2: STYLE IT! WORK IT! LOVE IT!

Believe it or not you can look stylish and fabulous without breaking the Bank. Notice how your favorite celebrity stylist looks fabulous all the time? Well they have personal stylists at their beck and call and an unlimited budget at their disposal. For the average woman looking fashionable can be a challenge. It is possible to look fabulous regardless of how much you spend. The key is to know your personal style, or figure out the style you would love to aspire to then find the wardrobe pieces that highlight it. Changing your style is not just physical, but emotional. Begin your journey of physical and emotional self-transformation by answering the following questions you can

Who are you as a person?

A woman's style is a reflection of who she is. Personal style depends on your age. Do you dress according to your age? It also depends on your occupation. Are you the modern woman who works in the corporate world? Are you a modest kindergarten teacher? Whatever you do can serve as a guide to what your personal style can be. It means you can go from office to happy hour by adding a few accessories to add some flair. What about your lifestyle? To describe my personal style it is classy-chic, casually elegant yet conservative. Heels can make any outfit look great, but worn in the wrong environment, will be uncomfortable.

Who inspires your style?

There are so many style icons around the world to choose from. Who you choose is up to your own discretion of course. However, it does not hurt to browse websites and magazines to emulate elements that you would like to incorporate in your own style and wardrobe. As I said before, you can't go wrong if you start simple.

What do you want to accomplish?

Change sometimes indicates new beginnings. It can also suggest moving to a new goal in your life. You may want to make that big career change. Therefore, your fashion goals and your life goals go hand in hand. Make a list to serve as a guide of the pieces you want to add to your wardrobe.

What do you have in your wardrobe?

This is a great place to start by assessing your current style. Look for anything that is ripped, stained, worn, too big or too small, and dispose of them. However, you may find some timeless pieces that could be accessorized. I say make a few changes and take baby steps. You do not need to make any drastic changes and fashion evolves. However, pick a few new things that could enhance what you already have.

The following are just a few examples of some key pieces that you can start with. They are not expensive yet I believe in quality over quantity.

To start how about some *luminous pearls*; at least two go-to *statement necklaces*, a go-to *handbag*, a *fabulous clutch* (or two) to complete a casual or formal look, a *classy watch*, a great pair of *diamond stud earrings*, which add flair to any outfit yet, and its not extravagant. In addition, having *fabulous drops* can take any outfit from drab to elegant. There was a time when I disliked necklaces and if you ask me why, well, I am still asking the same question every time I wear one. The rules are simple: wear studs with statement necklaces or small drops and wear longer drops without the necklace. There is just no going around it. I have seen women wear long drops, extravagant necklaces with dresses that have an embellished neckline. It is unnecessary as you want to enhance your natural beauty not suffocate it under glitz. The great thing is that no one is perfect and even many of your style icons have made a few styles hiccup here and there.

You can't go wrong with *black tank tops* to wear underneath your *blazers, cardigans* or *sheer tops* as well as a *black turtleneck* (timeless), *white tops, black pants*, and great *quality jeans*.

The *Little Black Dress* is like God's gift to women. There is no limit on how many you should have. Black dresses are fantastic to have because the color looks stately, timeless and gorgeous against your skin tone. With so many styles to choose from you could easily get overwhelmed. Find a simple, plain black dress (sleeveless is stunning!) to start with. Why? For the simple reason that you can accessorize it multiple ways and wear it over and over. In time you will find some more stylish black dresses. One shoulder dresses are still in; a trend that will not disappear any time soon. The more black dresses the better for you because they are timeless and are a fashion staple. The possibilities are endless, but a little black dress is effective.

The *pencil skirt* is another great staple, which can be worn casual or formal, not to mention they are extremely sophisticated. The pencil skirt is a great piece that can go from day to evening. I recommend starting with black, blue or both. A pencil skirt is quite ideal as you can pair it with different tops, and other accessories to create multiple looks. A great trench coat or pea coat is a great pick for those who live in the colder weather; this is essential, stylish and keeps off the harsh cold. Of course there are other alternatives you can find within your budget.

Black pumps-this is another classic staple for your closet to polish the look you are going for. Pick and choose the right one for you. Personally I love 'peep-toe' shoes and I wear them in black and nude. The fact is that shoe styles change and a pointed peep toe shows off your beautiful French pedicure depending on your preference. A critical accessory you will often forget is your *hair!* There is nothing wrong if you are not an expert at styling your hair or being able to afford treatments. Pace yourself and learn the correct steps based on your hair type. Avoid, as best as possible, gels, grease, heat, permanent colors that bleach the hair and holding sprays. Everyone has their own preference but a hair with movement looks much healthier than a hair with too much products. Your hair should always be well-groomed at all times. I will explore hair further in another chapter.

Just remember though, your best accessory yet is confidence: a great attitude and your billion-dollar smile!

Chapter 3: Enhance and Accentuate, But Don't Alter

Women have different body types. As such will need the right clothes to highlight them. The best thing to start with is a great fitting bra. Get measured for your right size and choose a fit, which will look flawless under a tight body shirt. Not only do you look and feel great, you are preventing future back and shoulder pains that could affect you later on in life. Visit your local department stores or you can check out Body by Victoria's Secret. It accentuates your natural curves; the quality is amazing and extremely comfortable. Finding the right bra can be a very painful journey for many women. However, don't despair. Make it a priority for the New Year.

If you are a full-figured woman who is pear-shaped it is wise to avoid horizontal stripes and big patterned clothing. Instead, draw attention to your upper body. This is the only time you are allowed to go for bright tops, scarves and shoulder pads. A shoulder pad adds the illusion of height and adds proportion to your body shape. Go for tailored and darker colors for your bottoms (pants, skirts, etc.). If you are of a more rounded shape go for empire waist dresses or tops, and tailored wide-legged pants. I do understand that many women are not as endowed as others and may be flat chest. However, do not despair. My suggestion is to opt for round neck tops, and add a bold statement necklace that will pull the eye away from your chest. On the other hand, women who are 'busty' usually have a problem finding the right tops. How about wearing scooped neckline tops and dresses that hug your chest appropriately? I will reiterate that a great fitting bra can help solve some of your bust issues whether you are big busted or flat chest.

Chapter 4: Get With The Glow!

People say beauty is only skin deep, but the importance of skin goes a lot deeper. The skin is an organ and like your internal organs, it must be protected and cared for. As we get older so too our skin ages and becomes thinner and drier. Be prepared for wrinkles, age spots, dark under-eye circles and large pores which tend to turn up like uninvited guests at a wedding. However, my job is to show you some fantastic natural ways to get the same glow that make up can provide. I have gotten numerous compliments on my skin and how much I am glowing. How did I do it? I started to become extremely careful about what I eat and put on my skin. For starters, I live in a tropical climate; therefore it is inevitable that skin care is my number one priority.

The glow I speak of is usually typical of pregnant women, but you too can have it.

Tip One-Water and Lemon

The way you start your day is important. The moment you wake up in the mornings, have a tall glass of water. This allows oxygen to flow through your cells and it will leave you feeling revived and energetic. You can also indulge in a cup of warm water with a drop of lemon juice. Lemon is powerful antioxidants, which help to boosts your immune system, and it is a great source of Vitamin C. While lemon is acidic on its own, inside our bodies it becomes alkaline. In short, an alkaline body is the key to good health. It also helps balance your weight by reducing your hunger cravings and it also helps with digestion. However, one of the most important benefits is that it gives you clear and beautiful skin while hydrating you. How amazing is that? It makes a world of difference and you will feel remarkable and happy for the rest of the day. I recommend you try this for a month and eventually it will become part of your daily routine.

Tip Two-Chewable Vitamin C

"Pop" Vitamins C's like they are going out of style. Having at least two in the mornings is a sure way to boost your immune system. A healthy immune system means clear skin and your hair and nails will grow. I absolutely love the chewable vitamins. You will like them if you dislike taking pills. It is important to note that you should not take more than the recommended dosage for the day. Too much Vitamin C can actually make you Vitamin C deficient. If you wish you can also eat the fruits or drink the juices that are rich in Vitamin C. Soon you will see your skin looking smoother and you are glowing.

Tip Three-The power of Aloe Vera

You simply can't go wrong by using Aloe Vera. Many people have even eaten the insides of the raw plant and gotten amazing results. I also know it leaves your hair very clean and shiny when used as a shampoo substitute. However, I use the Aloe Vera gel at nights and also in the mornings on my skin. You can check out your local drug stores for this 'miracle in a bottle' and use as much as you desire. Aloe Vera has no known side-effects. I apply this as a sunscreen substitute on days when it is cloudy or overcast. The oily residue of sunscreen on oily skin can be messy. However, wearing sunscreen is important because of the SPF ingredient.

Tip Four-Fruits and Veggies

What you put in your body does affect the way your skin looks. Sometimes it is best to eat meats sparingly and fill up on fruits and vegetables. If you are on a diet you can incorporate some organic foods such as green leafy vegetables, broccoli, carrots, tomatoes, lettuce, cucumbers, spinach, apples, bananas, grapes, melons and any others that you may like. The results? A healthy immune system and skins that glows for days!

Tip Five-Be Gentle With Your Skin

Avoid using harsh soaps on your face. Treat your face like a precious gem. When you wash your face use soaps that will not dry out your skin. A mild soap I can suggest is Dove, which leaves a thin film that locks in the moisture. Use warm water to wash and open the pores and cold water to close them and seal in the moisture. It is best to let your face air dry naturally. If you must use a towel it is best to pat your face dry. Leave your face a little damp so it can dry on its own then apply your moisturizer.

Tip Six-Massage

It is recommended that you brush your hair from root to tip and massage the scalp to allow blood and oxygen to circulate to your skin cells effectively. Similarly, you can massage your face muscles to stimulate blood flow, which will make your skin look flush and bright. These are just a few of many tips you can follow to get the natural glow. In the next section I will be providing some scrubs and masks you can make at home to help enhance that glow.

Chapter 5: Do-It-Yourself Natural Scrubs and Masks That Make Your Skin Glow!

As a little girl growing up I had acne problems. My mother took me to several Dermatologists, but after two weeks of using the soaps, my face would break out again. My brother suggested I used Aloe Vera as a facial mask so I did for about a month, cut out sweeteners from my diet, had plenty of water coupled with a sulfuric-based soap and I was able to control it. That was when I got curious about what else I could use and started to experiment with ripe Avocado, which I had in unlimited supply. I noticed how remarkably soft and refreshed it left my face feeling. Below I will share with you some of my personal favorite facial masks and scrubs. Before you begin using any of the tips below, there are some general scrub and mask procedures that you should follow. Pull your hair back and wash your face with warm water or steam with hot water to open your pores. Avoid the eye area at all times because it is very sensitive.

While others say rinse off with warm water I say rinse with cold water as you already opened your pores. Enjoy the results!

Coconut Milk and Egg White

In a small mixing bowl, add about 2 tablespoons of coconut powder milk along with 1 egg white. Add a few drops of water and use a small whisk to blend the ingredients to get a smooth paste. Wash your face with warm water to open the pores, use a clean towel to pat dry, but leave it damp. On a clean face apply the paste on your forehead, your cheeks, chin and nose. Avoid the eyelids at all times as it is a very sensitive area. Use a clean hand to move the paste on your cheeks in an upright motion so it sets well in your pores. Spread it over your forehead in a circular motion and finish by blending the rest over the other untouched areas. Your neck and chest is an extension of your face. Use the remaining paste in the bowl to apply to your neck and chest and if you feel adventurous, feel free to apply to your shoulders. Leave the paste to dry for at least 10-15 minutes. It can be up to 20 minutes depending on your schedule. Soon it will dry and your face will feel very stiff. Yes it may feel weird, but the results will be worth it. Rinse off your face with cold water to close the pores and locked in all the moisture you just infused in your skin. The coconut leaves your face feeling soft and the egg white functions as a collagen to tighten the pores and if you have any wrinkles it will reduce them.

Egg White, Honey and Lemon Juice Mask

Whisk 1 egg white until it becomes frothy; add 1 teaspoon of honey and 1 teaspoon of lemon juice. Apply and leave on for 15-20 minutes. The egg whites tighten the skin while the lemon juice lightens any discolorations and it disinfects. The honey is very soothing and nourishing for your skin.

Tomato Paste Mask

I swear by this mask that it is amazing. Blend 2 very ripe red tomatoes in a blender; add 1 teaspoon of lemon juice and 1 teaspoon of oatmeal until a paste is formed. Apply to skin for 10-15 minutes and rinse off with cold water (if you pre-washed your face with warm water before applying mask). A tomato contains a lot of vitamins, mineral and antioxidants and is a natural astringent which helps remove excess oils and refines your pores. It's one of the best I have used and the results are amazing. This is also the ultimate way to get your face glowing.

Banana and milk

The ultimate moisturizer, banana and cows milk leaves your face feeling smooth and refreshed. Blend 1 banana and approximately half cup of cow's milk in a blender or you can use a whisk. When it forms a paste, apply to pre-washed face and leave for 10-15 minutes. The smoothness of your skin is unbelievable and it leaves your face glowing!

- ## Facial Scrubs that make your face glow!

Lemons Juice, Honey and Brown sugar Scrub

Brown sugar smells divine and feels amazing on your skin as a scrub even by itself. Sugar is a natural glycolic acid and helps exfoliate dead, dry skin while the lemon juice brightens any discolorations. Add 1 teaspoon of lemon, 1 tablespoon of honey and 1 tablespoon of brown sugar. Massage into the skin and rinse. You will feel refreshed and your face feels extremely smooth.

Baking Soda Scrub

Baking soda is perfect for your everyday use. Simply add 3 teaspoon of baking soda to a small amount of water. Mix them into a paste and exfoliate in a circular motion. I love the feel of the fine grains as they move over my skin.

Oatmeal Scrub

This scrub has three benefits. It smoothes, tones and hydrates. Add 1 tablespoon of oatmeal and 1 teaspoon of lemon juice. Mix them into a paste and apply by gently massaging it into the skin.

Banana Scrub

This scrub smells delicious and is finely textured. Blend 1 ripe banana, 2 teaspoon of oats, and 1 teaspoon of milk and 1 teaspoon of honey. Apply to face and massage. As an added bonus you can leave it on your face to dry as a mask for 10-15 minutes. Rinse off with cold water.

These are just some of the amazing masks and scrubs you can make at home on your own. The ingredients can be found in your cupboard and quite inexpensive. They are made from natural and organic fruits and foods, which contain numerous vitamins and minerals, which are essential for skincare.

Chapter 6: Make-up: Less is more!

I hope you have tried at least one of my homemade masks and scrub. After that experience of treating your face, do you really want to clog up your pores with too much makeup? As a woman you will love to wear your makeup as it polishes the look you are going for. However, it is important to know when less is more. In addition, you can easily cause your face to break out if you sleep in your make up. I strongly advice to use a makeup remover to remove it, clean your face thoroughly and add a moisturizer. Even if you suffer from oily skin, you still need to use a moisturizer. Know what works for you and if you are in doubt, you should seek expert help. Sometimes you need to realize that less is more. If you must wear makeup, you must avoid clogging your pores with too much foundation. I can certainly understand that you may have blemishes and spots or discoloration. Obviously you will need makeup to create a more even skin tone. The one thing I can suggest is to treat the problem naturally. If it is beyond your control then you should seek the expert advice of your Dermatologist. It's perfectly acceptable to wear makeup while you are undergoing treatment for any facial issues. The best thing to use is a tinted moisturizer, which you can get from brands such as L'Oreal, Maybelline or MAC. Of course there are lower end ones that I am sure you can find at your local drug stores. Choose the best one for you, use a stipple brush and apply in a circular motion on your face. To eliminate the spots, try using a color corrector. Color correctors are very useful to treat severe skin issues and even discolorations. Hardly anyone has perfect flawless skin so it is great to even out hyper-pigmentation, redness and scarring in your complexion. It is best to have an expert assist you with this at best. From my understanding, if you have deep blue, purple circles or any bruising color, use a yellow tone corrector to even out your skin tone. It is best not to apply too much foundation on these areas to cover these flaws. Use the color corrector then apply your foundation with a foundation brush. I am not a professional or an expert, but what little I know I will share. I do wear makeup, but it is mineral based with SPF and applied very lightly so my pores can breathe. Makeup is supposed to enhance your most beautiful features not alter the way you look. It should not be that it appears you are wearing layers of it. You also owe it to yourself to work with lipstick shades that are closer to your lip color. Not everyone is Avant-garde as others. Do everything in moderation. I am a woman of color and while my skin tone allows me to wear bright shades, I ensure that my eye shadow is neutral with brighter lips or my lips is neutral with brighter shades of eye shadows. I love earth tones and bronze colors, but at times I do feel "adventurous". It will change depending on the look I am going for. Sometimes I do not feel like wearing any or I may choose to wear a simple winged liner look that looks just as good. If you would like tutorials on doing your makeup, there are thousands of videos on YouTube that you can watch. The videos are easy to follow and you are through the process.

Hair is the ultimate accessory!

I am a firm believer in enhancing your natural beauty instead of altering. One way to do so is styling your hair appropriate as the ultimate accessory. No look is ever complete without 'bombshell' hair. If you love curls, but are afraid of heat there are ways to get the same look without using a curling iron. One of the most effective ways is to use "flexi-rods." They are phenomenal. I always pull out the rods last when I am getting dressed to go out. For me, the rods give a better texture of curls and they last longer. If you are strapped for time and you must use a curling iron, curl your hair and immediately wrap it around the flexi-rod so it cools on it. It creates some amazing curls that look fabulous with any outfit. However, heat can damage your hair and block your efforts to grow your hair out. It took me five years to grow my hair out from two inches to fourteen inches. After applying too much heat to my hair it began to break and as a result I had to cut it off and start fresh. It was a hard decision but today I love the result. I am not advising you to cut off your hair. In fact, avoid "scissors happy" hair stylists. Sometimes the best treatments for "split ends" is to deep condition, use a leave-in conditioner and apply hair moisturizer. Finally, avoid bleaching and applying permanent color to your hair. Regardless of your hair type or race, adding too much chemicals to the shaft of the hair strips it of its natural oils and luster. The best thing to start with is a semi-permanent color after deep conditioning. If you must use permanent color, be sure to deep condition after and add plenty of hair lotion. Wash your hair at least once per week; then apply a semi-permanent color. Use a shampoo and conditioner specifically for color treated hair and one that hydrates and moisturizes. There are so many brands available to choose from so pick wisely.

Chapter 7: Love, Relationships And Heartbreak

Love yourself and know that you are amazing. You may feel that when it comes to love and relationships you are fighting a losing battle. Stop "fighting" and begin to fight for you. Have the courage to walk away from anything or anyone that is not contributing to your happiness. If you feel you do not have a choice, I say you always have a choice. No matter how devastating and hurtful the situation you are in may be, never allow bitterness to overcome you. Bitterness will eat away your insides and cause a flood of bad hormones to take over your body. Imbalance in hormones will certainly lead to depression. Depression is a door you do not want to open. Whenever you are feeling down, treat yourself to something wonderful or a new experience. Watch your circle of friends and be mindful of the persons who are not looking out for your best interests.

Fabulosity is you, but you have to believe it. Throw away the negatives and push yourself towards more positive systems of beliefs and ideas. Trust the process of life that you were meant to do amazing things for yourself and others. I believe you must empower yourself fully first to stand against an unpredictable world. The more positive energy you send out the more you attract positive people and opportunities. With this mind frame and belief, I truly believe that love will find you. It's always great to make plans, but accept that plans will change and you are capable of enjoying the process. Five years ago I was a student at University and I had completely devoted my time and life to succeeding in my studies. I had the option to date, but for some reason I pointedly told the individual that I do not see the relationship getting very far. Of course he did try to pursue me, but I knew "not all that glitters was gold." I had this vision of what real love was supposed to be and it certainly was not with that individual. I only wanted to focus solely on my education and considered relationships to be a "distraction" from my goals. Like you I had a plan. I did have a plan of graduating first, getting a job, meeting my future husband and getting married (in that order). Somehow without expecting it, my husband and I met at a time when we both wanted the same things in life. Things happen in a way you least expect it to because I met my husband while as a student. What many people do not know is that we were engaged for two years.

During that period we did encounter little challenges, but we never lost sight of our goals. I still smile about this sometimes and now I have been married for almost two years and together we have grown.

Everything in life is about patience. Nothing good ever comes from rushing. Wanting something big to happen now will not get you to where you are going any faster. However, make realistic goals and concentrate on achieving them. Life is about pursuing purpose. If you are single, these are the things you do to make it possible for someone else to meet you halfway. There is no need to rush, be patient. I do believe God is making your husband into a man before you meet him. Do you want someone to just love and make you feel validated or do you also want someone who will be your partner in everything. Wonderful things and people will come into your life when you least expect it. Focus on building your personal brand. I believe that you should respect yourself enough and love yourself no matter what. You have more power and capacity within you than you will probably use in your lifetime. You are beautiful, talented, amazing and simply the best at being you. Always be the best version of yourself and know that you deserve everything good in life. You deserve all the love and respect in the world. Know within yourself that you are worthy of all the good things in life. Soon enough you will realize that at some point you will have to let go of all the pointless drama and even the people who create it. Surround yourself with people who will make you laugh so hard that you forget the bad and focus solely on the good. After all, life is too short to be anything, but happy.

Love yourself. Be authentic. Be true to yourself. Judy Garland once said: "Always be a first rate version of yourself instead of a second rate version of somebody else". If you can live by this statement, you will realize that there is no such thing as living in someone else's shoes. The only shoes you can occupy are your own. If you aren't being yourself, you aren't truly living, but you merely exist. Value yourself, but be financially smart. Be creative and resourceful and avoid putting yourself in debts. If you experience heartbreak it is just a way of breaking you to make you twice as strong. It is quite fine to feel hurt and angry. I say embrace the process and understand that the person was only in your life for a reason and a season. He or she fulfilled his or her purpose and moved on. Ask yourself what lessons you have learned from the experience. I hope one of those lessons is not that you will never love or trust again. Wrong! You will love and trust again. You just have to have faith and believe. If you are religious or spiritual you have to believe that God's timing is everything. You biggest challenge will be how to overcome the biggest enemies you have created within yourself: hate, anger, bitterness, feelings of humiliation and the biggest one revenge. You should not waste time on revenge. Anyone who has hurt you will eventually find his or her own karma. It does not mean you are going to sit around waiting for something bad to happen to him or her. It means that at some point he or she will encounter a situation that will make them ponder on the mistakes made in the past (whether to you or someone else). Forgive immediately. You deny yourself a life free of anger and hate by holding unto resentment. You have to ask yourself for forgiveness for any hateful thoughts and ideas that come into focus. Finally, forgive those who hurt you. Nothing annoys them more. Just remember that the emotional roll-a-coaster of your life will not let up until you can appreciate you for you.

Chapter 8: Secrets to a Happy Marriage: Confessions Of A Newlywed

Marriage is a beautiful institution, but never take it for granted. Growing up I always heard people complain of various issues that affect their marriages. I've listened to women give details of how much they became calculated and suspicious of their partners. There are so many things that can erode the foundations of a good marriage and sadly many couples fall into this trap. After I got married, the question posed to me the most was "How is married life?" My answer is always simple: " It's everything I expected." There are no surprises!

The truth is marriage is not for everyone. You should ensure you understand the real reasons for getting married. You and your partner should love and respect each other in order to have a healthy marriage. Make sure before you walk down that isle you have no reservations and you are certain that this is the right step for you. Having unrealistic expectations will cause a breakdown in communication. As a consequence, it will affect your marriage.

As for me, I am happily married. My husband and I are best friends and we can communicate effortlessly. We support each other in all aspects of our life. The love and bond we share is quite powerful and impenetrable. As time goes by we embrace both the internal and external changes that affects our lives. We also thrive on excluding 'third parties' that try to cause disruption in our lives. We are mindful of our circle and very aware of those who would want to cause some measure of friction for their own personal gain. I say this because there are people who do not understand the bond between a couple in a relationship. They make attempts to project their own unhappiness on you. Your husband is your best friend first and everyone one else comes after. A very key element of marriage is RESPECT. Yes. Your husband should have your complete and utter respect and he should do the same. I respect my husband for several reasons because he never compromises on his values. Whatever he says that is exactly what he means and I can trust him completely.

While celebrating our first anniversary of being married we met three American couples. One was married for 36 years, one for 17 years and another 15 years. There we were; a table of strangers who all began to share our thoughts on marriage. The husbands all 'ganged up' on the wives and agreed that they just said 'yes dear' to everything. It was quite amusing as I listened to them make light of the situations they experienced, but behind it all was a deep respect unlike none other. The overall conclusion was that marriage is about compromise. That goes for any relationship. Marriage is a beautiful experience.

You may be turned off from the idea of getting married. Perhaps you have listened to the horror stories of other people and what you have observed, you can't even begin to fathom the notion. The truth is you live in society where you are taught that marriage is supposed to be impermanent. However, I was born to parents who were married so it was not a question for me. That was the only choice I knew as a child. Of course you are entitled to your own choice and may choose not to be married, simply because you don't think it is necessary. Still, it is not something to be feared. You may fear losing your identity. In fact, your partner is your other half and is there to support you in everything. In my marriage, it has even brought me closer to God. Do not be afraid to pray together and keep thanking God for all his blessings. Yes. God is a vital part of our household. A family that prays together stays together and that is great. Once you put God and keep him in the middle you should be fine. If you are a newlywed or you are getting ready to tie the knot, just remember that marriage is what you make it. Life is what you make it.

Chapter 9: Nothing is as Sexy as a Woman With Confidence

Be so confident in yourself that when you walk into a room no one has to second-guess who you are. There is nothing more attractive than confidence. Your confidence should be the result of knowing your worth, achieving your goals and having fun while doing it. Once you see your own beauty, so will everyone else. Confidence is how you speak, but be mindful of what you say. There is a fine line between ego and confidence. Ego is a form of madness. I can understand you have worked hard to overcome most of the hurdles in your life. No one is perfect and no one expects you to be. You can't expect to inspire someone if you come across as being condescending. What you don't know is that the person you are trying to impress was already impressed. Confidence is humility. Humility is not a weakness, but strength. Know that everyone occasionally suffers from a lack of confidence; even the person you're trying so hard to impress. I don't believe anyone has the right to discount others. I believe in helping others and offer genuine advice. I love when someone turns his or her passion into reality. Living your own passion could eventually have you employing those who once said you could not do it

Confidence is everything. Make your next move boldly. One of the most attractive things you should have is a confident presence. Being comfortable in your own skin is key. Take care of your physical and emotional self and wear comfortable clothing you like. When in doubt, simplicity is the ultimate form of sophistication. As I mentioned before: less is more. The way you speak is also an important factor in demonstrating confidence. Trying to impress someone by being too verbose can work against you if it isn't the natural way that you speak. Some of the most intelligent women out there use simple words, but make big statements. Be your own trailblazer, and dream big. Stop worrying about what others will think of you, and just be yourself. Confidence is simply about being comfortable in your own skin. Trust your instincts and be decisive. Watch your circle because there will be "friends" who will try to shake your confidence. Do not allow anyone to place his or her unhappiness on you. Celebrate your individuality. Love yourself and face your fears. Take care of your mind, body and soul. Know your worth! Do not settle for less that you are worth! You deserve

all the good in the world. Do things to
make yourself happy so others can love
you too. Self-love is the greatest. Be bold
and confident. Be the beautiful sexy you.

Chapter 10: Whip That Body in Shape: Effective Exercise Programs & Routines That Works

I am a sports enthusiast, but working out and eating healthy is part of my lifestyle. I do not believe you need to go to the gym to lose weight and get fit. Quite frankly I will take the fresh outdoors over a hot sweaty gym. The last time I went to the gym the instructor had me lifting weights while my cardio was being neglected. I decided to stop and work out on my own. I wanted to lose the weight first then tone up. By weight I do not mean fat as I am quite athletic, but I do know when it's time to burn some calories. After the first month of working out on my own, I decided that Gyms are a waste of time and money. Your body is the ultimate sculpting machine. I will share with you a list of simple exercise routines and exercise programs that can tone your body in just one week. Exercise workouts raises your heart rate. You also burn more claories.

Effective Exercise Programs & Routines That Work

My favorite and recommended exercise programs that you can do from the comfort of your home are:

- *Total Body Sculpt (Gilad)*
- *Bodies in Motion (Gilad)*
- *Zumba*
- *Ten minutes cardio workout videos on YouTube.*
- *Beginners Yoga that is much slower. It is great to tighten your abdominals.*

Here are some effective routines to help sculpt your body:

Cardio

Mild Stretching-This help to get the muscles warmed up and loosened for more intensive workouts.

Power Walking-Very effective and you can burn as much calories as you would from jogging.

High Knees-I recommend these if you do not want to go jogging outside. It's like running in the same spot.

Swimming-This helps with you're breathing and tones your entire body.

Jumping jacks-I recommend at least twenty to twenty five that helps you *burn calories and work out the whole body.*

Push-ups-Attempt at least ten and increase by five thereafter.

Squats-If you want nice shapely thighs and a firmer posterior, then relax and do at least fifty every two to three days. Do what you can manage.

Abdominals

Bicycle Crunches-A great workout for your upper and lower abs as well as your obliques.

Abdominal Twist-Great for working your obliques!

Leg raise-This works the lower abs that are sometimes hardest to target.

Basic Exercise Equipment To Have At Home

Two must have exercise equipment are *Perfect Sit-ups* and *Dumbbells*. *Perfect Sit-ups* is very good because as you raise your body from the floor by holding firmly to the handles it helps you to maximize your efforts. When you hear a click, it means that you have achieved maximum efficiency in the exercise movement. The *Dumbbells* are excellent for toning your arms, chest muscles, thighs and legs. Notice how First Lady Michelle Obama has "obamamise" her fabulous arms. The best *Dumbbell* weights to have are five pounds and if you are fairly advance ten pounds. Always hydrate your body. Remember, water is your best friend. Eat more whole grains, fruits and vegetables. Again, water is your best friend. Drink it like its "going out of style." Have a glass of Gatorade immediately after working out; it replaces the electrolytes you lost. Your body needs to repair itself quickly. Do not try to lose weight by eating less than your expected daily calorie intake. If you are a woman between 19-30 years old you will need approximately 2000 calories per day. I can understand if you intake 1800, but not if you intake 1200. That is almost half of your calorie intake for the day, which means you have sent your body into starvation mode. The key to weight loss is balance. You cannot lose weight without balancing your diet and exercise. There are so many "experts" on the topic who said that you can lose weight without exercise. It is not healthy to "lose ten pounds in two weeks *fast.*" Sacrificing nutrition for exercise or exercise for nutrition will result in decreased health. The best option is to "meet the need" and strike that balance. I can suggest a great App that can help you record your weight loss progress, which is *My Fitness Pal.* You are required to create a profile and log your daily food intake and calories. It is able to calculate how many calories you need based on your age, height, gender and weight. This is just one that I can suggest as I am sure there are a lot of free Apps you can download for personal use. I sincerely hope these tips were helpful to you!

Author Bio

I am a multi-talented and happy young woman who has a passion for writing and inspiring people and hold a Bachelor of Arts Degree in English Literatures & a minor in Cultural Studies with very high honors and hope to change thoughts and lives of people with my books. I am happily married to my loving husband who is also my best friend. Together we have achieved and continue to motivate each other to fulfill our goals. While I enjoy writing, I also enjoy traveling and experiencing different cultures and meeting new people. Currently I am working on my first novel about growing up in Jamaica.

THANK YOU FOR READING!

The purpose of this book is to inspire young women who has ever struggled to find their true purpose in life and who now wants to live a life of strength, promises, purpose, power and potential. The message is powerful yet simple: you can begin to change your life and your future by accepting that you are perfect inside and outside. However, to be successful you should be bold, fearless and empowered. If after reading this book you are still looking for an extra "push", my others books *Ten Life Changing Lessons* and *The Perks Of A Positive Attitude: A Practical Guide To Happiness And Success* will certainly give you the tools and inspiration to pursue your purpose. I believe in celebrating life and accept each day with gratitude and love. Thank you for reading my book. I hope you found it helpful with practical tips and advice that you can use to become a healthier, happier you.

Printed in Great Britain
by Amazon